D0829936

improve sleep

20 QUICK TECHNIQUES

*with 3 extra solutions
for jet lag*

KATRIN SCHUBERT, MD

Hazelden
Publishing

Hazelden Publishing
Center City, Minnesota 55012
hazelden.org/bookstore

Library of Congress Cataloging-in-Publication Data

Names: Schubert, Katrin, 1960- author.
Title: Improve sleep : 20 quick techniques with 3 extra
    techniques just for jet lag / Katrin Schubert, MD.
Description: Center City, Minnesota : Hazelden
Publishing, [2017] | Series: 5-minute first aid for the mind
Identifiers: LCCN 2016057798 | ISBN 9781616497224
    (paperback)
Subjects: LCSH: Sleep—Popular works. | Sleep disorders
    —Alternative treatment—Popular works. |
    Insomnia—Alternative treatment—Popular works. |
    Self-care, Health—Popular works. | BISAC: HEALTH
    & FITNESS / Sleep & Sleep Disorders. | SELF-HELP/
    Personal Growth / General.
Classification: LCC RA786 .S38 2017 | DDC
    616.2/09—dc23
LC record available at https://lccn.loc.gov/2016057798

21 20 19 18 17   1 2 3 4 5 6

Cover design: Kathi Dunn, Dunn + Associates
Interior illustrations: Marty Harris Illustration
Author photo: Deb Stagg
Development editor: Vanessa Torrado
Production editor: Heather Silsbee

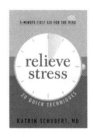
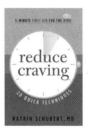

Dedicated to the power
of a good night's sleep

CONTENTS

Introduction

"The best sleep is the sleep you get before midnight," my grandmother used to tell me as she tucked me into bed. She would elaborate that I would stay healthier, wiser, and more youthful if I heeded her advice and prioritized an early bedtime hour. Those words of sage advice were given in the early days of my childhood—well before teenage parties, working night shifts, and burning the midnight oil poring over books. And it was *long* before my young children woke me up nightly, leaving me with a "new normal" of disrupted sleep. It was also before my routines were determined by my work schedule and personal concerns kept my mind preoccupied at night.

Certainly, my story will be familiar to many readers. Add to the common scenarios of our everyday lives our ever-growing love affair with watching movies, bingeing on TV shows, and being attached to our various electronic devices, and it is safe to say few of us are following my grandmother's advice.

We know we have to get up in the morning to tend to our daily routine, but we end our days with very late nights—even though research has confirmed my grandmother's wisdom. If we go to sleep well before midnight and get a full night of sleep—rather than getting the same amount of sleep starting after midnight—it has been shown that our bodies and minds will stay healthier, and we will feel happier and more rested.

How did we get here? What has changed from the end of the twentieth century to our current place in the twenty-first?

Many of us seem to have lost our healthy sleep patterns. Gone are the days of rising with the sun, working hard physically during the day, and going to sleep at sundown. We are staying awake longer and doing different types of activities during our waking time. Over the past decades, we have come to work harder and longer hours. Our stress levels have pushed our nervous systems into overdrive, and we find it more challenging to find a balance between work and leisure. Ever-present cutbacks at work have loaded more tasks on our shoulders, and our minds are busier than ever, keeping us from thinking about or finding relaxation time. Then, with the expansion of the world around us through TV and the Internet, we are instantly connected to the latest news and the newest movies, and our friends are just a few keystrokes away. Late-night mental and electronic stimulation is keeping our bodies and minds very busy and awake.

Adults aren't the only ones to acquire these new habits. Kids are growing up in a different world too. Children are overloaded with what we tend to think of as "leisure" activities. Oftentimes, between extra-curricular activities and their normal school day, many children end up with a demanding schedule that is the equivalent of a "work day" that is longer than that of many adults. With the increased mental activity and expectations that kids face, they are robbed of the sense of relaxation required to maintain healthy patterns for rest and sleep. Fewer children now play outdoors, exploring their neighborhoods with friends. Without such habits, children find themselves to be constantly uptight and alert rather than learning to relax, explore, and savor the moment. Whether they live in the city or the country, many kids rarely get out into nature, which is vital to a child's development. We need to establish a connection with nature for our kids to stay mentally and spiritually healthy. In the same way that we grown-ups have come to indulge our stresses in a streaming binge or late-night social media browsing, our kids are doing the same. Endlessly playing computer games affects their sleep routines—and more. Many a time have I found my children asleep in their beds with laptops or cell phones beside their pillows. This new normal is something we're all experiencing—young and old(er). What is it doing to us?

For all of us, at any age, a chronic lack of sleep affects our mental, emotional, and physical health. The evolution of our daily routine across the past three to four decades may have occurred slowly enough that we've had the opportunity to adjust somewhat to these taxing patterns; however, our bodies, minds, and relationships are paying the price of chronic overdrive.

The long-term disruption of sleep patterns has left many people experiencing fatigue, a persistent feeling of "mind fog," and a general sense of difficulty that creeps into their relationships and daily lives.

No wonder, then, that the consequences of chronic sleep deprivation have been in the public eye recently. Research indicates that our immune systems, as well as our personal and work relationships, are affected by fatigue. According to a recent study by the U.S. Centers for Disease Control and Prevention, 35 percent of American adults do not get seven hours of sleep per night. This pattern is associated with an increase in heart disease, diabetes, stroke, and other illnesses.

As a society of people experiencing a chronic lack of sleep, we have seen a negative impact on many aspects of our lives. There is even a noticeable impact for businesses, as insufficient sleep reduces job satisfaction and increases unethical behavior, work injuries, cyberloafing, and whittling away the workday. It's hard to be productive when it is difficult to pay focused attention. Our society's chronic sleep problem has grown to such a degree, and affected work performance so much, that some companies have a "pay for sufficient sleep" policy. Notably, the insurance company Aetna pays their employees a little extra for achieving twenty consecutive days of seven hours of sleep—a great investment that is paying high dividends by improving the work-life balance and productivity of their employees.

A number of North American companies, notably Google, Zappos, Ben & Jerry's, Facebook, and The Huffington Post, have gone to the extent of offering their employees sleep rooms, where they are permitted to catch up on sleep at work. In some cases, the individual sleeping "pods" get reserved in twenty-minute intervals and are booked well in advance. While it's a great benefit, this also indicates that many employees have simply lost touch with wholesome sleep patterns. We may have forgotten the principles of healthy sleep patterns to such a degree that our employers believe they need to intervene on both our behalf and theirs. So what are the solutions?

Fortunately for us, there is much we can do to improve our sleep. Starting here and now.

In this book, you will find various techniques that will help you start to think about rest and sleep differently and reestablish healthy sleep patterns, as well as many useful self-help tools to call on for insomnia. Finally, you'll find a few trip-saving techniques that will enable you to reset your inner body and mind clock, known as your "circadian rhythm," when you are traveling and experiencing jet lag.

I encourage you to try them all and then pick your favorites, making them part of your everyday routine. There's a connection between great sleep, managed stress levels, and a healthy life. If you like the techniques in this book, there are other books in the 5-Minute First Aid for the Mind series that you might find helpful. *Relieve Stress* and *Reduce Craving* have many effective techniques that can support a great night's sleep as well.

* * *

How to Use This Book

This book is designed to empower you, the reader, to discover and practice self-help techniques that support a deep, sound sleep. By reading this book and trying the exercises described, you can help yourself improve the quality of your sleep, alleviate the many forms of insomnia, or avoid the pitfalls of jet lag.

Ideally, you would read the entire book and then try each technique a few times to find the ones that work best for you. Becoming familiar with the techniques will enable you to apply them on the spot, whenever you need them, even when you don't have this book handy for reference.

Alternatively, maybe you do not have time to read the entire book right now. Maybe you are eager to try a technique or two right away. This book, like all the books in the 5-Minute First Aid for the Mind series, allows and encourages you to do exactly that: open up the book, leaf through the pages, and apply the techniques most appealing to you. You may decide to try other techniques later, as your needs change.

This book is made up of four parts, three of which contain techniques for different purposes. The first part focuses on learning or reestablishing healthy sleep patterns that were either never learned or may have been lost over time. In that part of the book, you will find information on what it takes to get a good night's sleep, establish a sleep routine, and recover a state of increased well-being by allowing your body's natural sleep rhythm to take hold.

The second part of this book has numerous techniques that help with insomnia. Truth is, insomnia can be a challenge to treat because its causes vary. When it comes to insomnia, it really is best to read through everything. Try all of the techniques, find what resonates and works for you, and then pick your favorites. The techniques can be combined with one another and repeated as often as you wish or need. All of the techniques I have included in this book have been used by my clients and friends for many years. It is worth pointing out that my own sleep issues led me to explore these techniques over the years, and I have called upon the tools in this book many times myself. I find them very helpful.

The third part is meant for the traveler. If you find yourself moving between time zones, you will need something to help alleviate jet lag. As a seasoned flyer myself, I have come to rely on these techniques many times—they are now invaluable to me whenever I know I need to adjust to time changes. The techniques for managing jet lag will help you adjust your circadian rhythm in less time, which alleviates the effects of jet lag, such as fatigue, mental fogginess, and feeling under the weather mentally, emotionally, and physically.

Finally, the fourth part of this book will give you an overview of the theories behind the modalities included in this book. Read this part to learn about how and why these techniques help many people get a better night's sleep.

As with any self-help tools, this book and the techniques within it are meant to help you along on your path of life. The information in this book is not a substitute for adequate health care. Rather, this book is meant to work alongside regular office visits and other professional assistance you may be receiving.

As these techniques offer a complementary approach, they may result in you requiring less medication and/or less frequent visits to your health care providers.

May you find your way to perfect well-being through sound sleep.

• • •

Part I:

Techniques for Creating Wholesome Sleep Patterns and Habits

A FEW EASY INTERVENTIONS will help reset your body's patterns for sleep time and wake time. The results will very likely make you feel more alert during the day. Research shows us that our immune and hormonal systems work more effectively when our bodies and minds are well rested. We are able to make smarter decisions when we aren't experiencing chronic stress and sleep deprivation.

Developing healthy sleep habits will reestablish your own natural circadian rhythm (everyone's is different) and will balance your melatonin levels. Melatonin is the body's sleep hormone. Without enough of it, our sleep patterns are unbalanced.

Establishing a healthy sleep routine is the first step in regaining natural sleep patterns. A sleep routine has the added benefit of bringing a level of awareness and mindfulness to how you approach your overall sleep health. Like any routine, it can help you be more grounded, happy, and aware as you approach improving the quality of your sleep to improve the quality of your life.

It may take a little effort initially to reset your "sleep thermostat"; however, after a short while you'll find that your routine has become nothing less than second nature.

• • •

The Secrets to a Good Night's Sleep

These suggestions from the sages of good sleep support a great night's sleep by building healthy sleep patterns that improve your overall sense of well-being. Follow these principles and, before you know it, you'll be saying that you are "so good at sleeping, you can do it with your eyes closed."

1. **Get at least twenty minutes of natural sunlight each day.** Light exposure during the day helps your body follow a normal sleep-and-wake cycle. Natural sunlight regulates your body's production and release of melatonin, the hormone that is excreted at night to induce the natural sleep cycle.

2. **Exercise (even a little) on a daily basis. Get out there and move!** It goes a long way to make you feel more relaxed and ready for your z's. Going for a walk, riding a bicycle, or getting to the gym for even twenty minutes a day will make a huge difference.

3. **Reduce the amount of fluids you drink in the evening.** Drinking water throughout the day is important for your body's health. Consuming liquids later in the evening can disrupt your sleep. You will feel more rested in the morning if you do not have to get up at night to answer nature's call. Everyone hears that they should drink more water throughout the day—and you should. But be mindful of *when* you are drinking that water. If you are consuming liquids late in the day and you find yourself unable to sleep through the night because you are regularly getting up to empty your bladder, then you might have found an easy way to improve the quality of your sleep.

4. **Reduce your exposure to any light source with a white or blue hue at least two hours before bedtime.** This means that for the best night's sleep, when it is getting close to bedtime, you need to trade in the time you spend in front of a screen for something like time spent with a good, old-fashioned book. Screens on TVs, laptops, and smartphones emit the types of light that will keep you up. Instead of staring at a screen, try unwinding with

relaxation or breathing exercises, soft and relaxing music, or just by spending time with your loved ones. Bright white-blue lights keep us wired! So avoid them close to bedtime. (Technique 3, titled Sleepy Blues and Amber Dreams, provides more detail on the importance of avoiding these lights.)

5. **Limit caffeine.** We are all aware of the invigorating effects of caffeine. But caffeine breaks down very slowly in the body, so coffee, tea, and caffeinated soft drinks can keep us up for hours. It is best to stop consuming caffeine around midafternoon if you want a good night's sleep. Only about 50 percent of the caffeine you consume is cleared out of your body in about five to seven hours. That means five hours after having a cup of coffee, your body is still holding on to half the caffeine you consumed. Here's an example of just how long it can take our bodies to process caffeine: a nursing newborn who receives caffeine from its mother's milk needs a whopping 97.5 hours to break down just *half* of the caffeine that it has absorbed from its mother!

The caffeine contained in chocolate can disrupt your sleep as much as having a caffeinated drink.

For example, I have noticed repeatedly that a dark chocolate dessert after dinner will keep me awake for hours. At times, a delicious chocolate dessert compels me to test (once again) whether I can get away with the little indulgence and still get a good night's sleep. So far, the result is always the same. If I indulge a little in the dark chocolate, I pay the price later with lack of sleep.

Paradoxically, there are some people who have a cup of coffee to induce sleep. I remember an elderly lady whose antidote to insomnia was getting out of bed and making herself a nice cup of coffee. With her cup of coffee consumed, she'd go back to bed for a sound sleep. I have a friend named Inge who tells me that a little dark chocolate at bedtime helps her sleep soundly. The point is to figure out what works *for you.* You will know how your body reacts to caffeine by observing its aftereffects. Maybe caffeine stimulates you; perhaps it doesn't. If you are one of the lucky few who can have a cup of coffee and fall right asleep, know that these reverse reactions to a substance are called "paradox reactions" and are known to both pharmacists and doctors. Get to know how *your* body reacts to caffeine. If it is keeping you up, then limit its consumption to earlier in the day.

6. **Take magnesium!** Magnesium can help you sleep in so many ways. It helps relax your muscles and your brain. While adding a magnesium supplement to your routine can be very helpful, so is just mindfully adding some magnesium-rich foods to your diet. Almonds, cashews, pumpkin seeds, leafy green vegetables, avocados, and bananas all contain high levels of this vital mineral. Another great way to expose your body to magnesium late in the day and get ready for rest is by adding Epsom salts to your bath. Epsom salts, which has magnesium as a main ingredient, allows your body to absorb this important mineral as you soak and relax in the tub. Add some Epsom salts to your bathwater, and you'll be relaxing your muscles and balancing your magnesium levels in no time.

7. **Keep cortisol levels low.** Your body makes a stress hormone called cortisol. High stress levels elevate our cortisol levels. High levels of cortisol in our bodies keep us awake because cortisol's release is a way our bodies enable alertness. As night

approaches, keep your cortisol levels managed by reducing your overall stress levels. Maybe that means not listening to the news, watching thrillers, or tackling disagreements toward the end of the day. You can't drift off into dreamland if your body is full of cortisol.

8. **Pick a special night ritual.** A relaxing bath works wonders to help your mind and body unwind. Sliding between your sheets after a warm bath will make you sink into your pillow and go to sleep more easily. Regularly reading a book or some poetry, using some relaxation exercises, listening to soft music, or meditating for a few minutes at the end of the day can make all the difference in telling your body it is time for sleep. Rituals can become a pattern that your body relies on as a signal for better sleep.

9. **Catch a catnap.** Fatigue will stop you from sleeping well at night. A short rest or nap will rejuvenate you and give you enough energy to finish your day. Researchers and nap aficionados recommend naps of no longer than twenty minutes; otherwise, you may feel groggy afterward.

Establish Great Sleep Ambiance

Healthy patterns and practices may be the bedrock of great sleep, but following these tips for creating great "sleep ambiance" in your home and bedroom is important for a comprehensive and regular routine:

1. **Sleep in the dark.** A completely dark room may help you get sound, uninterrupted sleep. The sleep-inducing hormone melatonin is released at dusk and during the night. Being exposed to lights, especially the ones that have a blue hue, will disrupt melatonin's release and therefore disrupt your ability to sleep soundly. If you frequently wake at night to make a jaunt to the bathroom, consider getting a dim red or orange light to lead your way rather than bright white or blue lights.

2. **Turn it all off!** Shutting off electricity and any electromagnetic fields in your bedroom allows your body to rest. You may have noticed how much better you feel when fluorescent lights are turned off after you have been exposed to them for a while. The same holds true for wireless Internet, cordless phones, and any electric and electronic devices. Many physicians understand that people heal

faster and more efficiently when the wireless Internet is shut off at night. Some specialists are of the opinion that anyone suffering from a chronic illness will only be able to truly heal if the wireless connections are shut off during the night. Turning off your electronic devices and wireless Internet might be the key to rest.

3. **Clear it out!** Clear your bedroom of TVs and computers, as well as bright white and blue lights (or install dimmable ones). Ideally, the ambiance in your bedroom invokes relaxation and has no electronic equipment.

4. **Find your perfect temperature.** Keeping your room cool but your bed warm can help you sleep. If your bedroom tends to be very cool, warming your bed with an electric blanket or heating pad can help you relax when you crawl into bed. Please make sure to turn it off and remove it when you get into bed, as having an electric current in your bed is not good for healthy sleep. Research has shown that it takes *much longer* to fall asleep when one is even just slightly cold in bed; however, breathing cool air *supports* your sleep.

5. **Comfort is key!** Needless to say, a proper mattress and pillow allow for a sound sleep. If you can fully relax into your cozy, comfortable, and supportive bed, you will sleep more soundly.

6. **Safety first!** Make sure you feel safe where you sleep. If you have any concerns about disruption, lock your door. You may feel more relaxed. A heavy blanket or body pillow can add to your sense of coziness.

• • •

TECHNIQUE 2

Create a Sleep Routine

Now that you've spent some time reading about different tactics you can integrate into your day-to-day routine to improve your sleep quality, here is an example of a healthy before-bed relaxation strategy. By developing a larger sleep routine that brings together all of the insights you just learned, you can start to count on a better-quality sleep night after night. Try following this routine, or tweak it to fit your lifestyle.

HOW TO BUILD A ROUTINE

1. **Set a bedtime.** Understanding how many hours you need to sleep to feel rested helps you establish a set time for going to bed. Creating a healthy sleep pattern with a regular bedtime can help you get enough sleep and promotes better long-term rest.

2. **Start shutting down.** Turn off your electronic devices one to two hours before your desired bedtime. If you are going to read before bed, you may want to pick up a printed book instead of a digital one.

3. **Create a restful environment.** Listen to soothing music or an audiobook. Turn down the lights. Start creating a dreamscape to surround you that supports relaxation.

4. **Unwind.** Run yourself a bath or take a hot, relaxing shower. Tend to yourself. Taking care of your body can help you feel better and improve your sleep.

5. **Focus on your needs.** About half an hour before your official bedtime, try one of the exercises in part 2 of this book to help address any of the underlying issues preventing you from sleeping better.

6. **Count your blessings!** About fifteen minutes before bedtime, make your way to bed, find your gratitude journal (see Technique 4), and add a few lines or paragraphs to it.

7. **Drift off.** At your ideal time, shut off your lights, lie down, and drift off.

8. **Need a little extra help?** If fifteen to twenty minutes go by and you are having trouble falling asleep, you may want to try a breathing exercise (such as Techniques 18 and 19) or Betty Erickson's Sleep Induction method (Technique 15), described later in this book.

TECHNIQUE 3

Sleepy Blues and Amber Dreams

Our current age of technology has brought us many benefits. Tools for conducting business, consuming both local and global news, and connecting with our family and friends anywhere in the world are within our reach at any given moment. We are more productive and in touch with people than we have ever been before. We love the newest devices and the miraculous things they can do—most of the time. We also know that every life-changing invention casts a shadow. Apart from the detrimental effects our devices can have on our relationships and work, we now know that the bright white or blue hue of TV screens and LED lights has a systemic effect on our bodies and our health. It has been said that the average person actually needs an additional thirty minutes of sleep each day. That's usually because not only are we not sleeping enough, but the quality of sleep we are getting is not good enough.

What do you commonly do before bedtime? Are you watching TV or checking e-mails and text messages? If so, your routine may be full of common sleep hindrances. The blue light emitted from TV, computer, phone, and tablet screens stimulates a "daytime" response in our circadian rhythms, fooling our brains into believing it is time to be awake. It interferes with the secretion of our healthy sleep hormone, melatonin, which prepares us to fall and stay asleep. While it is highly recommended that you turn off your electronic devices two hours before bedtime, and I mention taking that step in the previous technique, the reality is that this piece of advice is not practical for many people in our society. After working during the day, preparing dinner, tending to our children or loved ones, and completing homework and chores, our evening hours often become the quiet time we rely on to read the day's news online, check our latest e-mails or text messages, or catch up with our circle of friends and family on social media.

Research has revealed that while we're trying to fall asleep, the white-blue lights given off by our screens not only disrupt our nervous systems but also reduce the amount of time we spend in the important

REM (dream) stage of sleep. Folks who read their bedtime stories on electronic devices feel less rested than people who read paper books. There's a sense of ongoing time seduction when we end our day on a device. While you might feel compelled to read *just a little longer* on your electronic blue-light-emitting device, remember that you are shortening your actual time spent asleep, as well as reducing your resting dreamtime, which affects your sense of well-being the next day. In other words, both quality and quantity of sleep are affected by our love affair with our e-tools.

Newer computers and other electronic devices have a nighttime mode that turns their screens amber rather than bright white, and many apps are available for download to help us improve our z's by reducing a significant portion of the blue light emitted by our devices. After all, it may not be the exciting news or messages from your friends that you are reading late at night that are robbing you of your sleep—it might just be the blue light that is shining on you before you head to sleep. While it might sound extreme to the average person, many computer geeks like to wear amber-toned glasses at night while they continue working or playing on their computers. The amber tones shut out the white-blue light frequencies that wake us up.

Now that we've talked about light-exposure habits that might be keeping you up at night, let's talk about how you might not be getting enough light at other times of the day. Daytime exposure to full-spectrum light (which includes the white-blue hues we've just talked about) is a rather different story.

Spending time outside during daylight hours is very helpful to a great night's sleep, as bright, full-spectrum daylight sets our internal clock and allows our circadian rhythms to remain intact. Exposure to full-spectrum light during the day, and the resulting strong and healthy circadian rhythm, makes us more alert, mindful, and productive—a pretty desirable effect to have during the day! If you work away from daylight for most of the day, then a walk at lunchtime, early in the morning, or right after work can make a significant difference when it comes to getting sufficient sleep at night. For those working night shifts, life and sleep seem upside down. Shift workers who wear tinted glasses that block out blue light for the last couple of hours of their work shift have been shown to experience a more sound sleep after work.

TIPS FOR ADJUSTING YOUR LIGHT EXPOSURE
AT THE END OF THE DAY

Take these steps to help ensure that lights aren't affecting your sleep.

1. Install night-lights with amber-toned light bulbs.

2. Use dimmer switches in your bedroom and bathrooms.

3. Shut down your e-readers and devices at least one to two hours before going to sleep.

4. Shut out street and car lights by using light-blocking curtains.

5. Remove all electronic devices from your bedroom.

6. Use the night setting, when available, on your computer or electronic device.

7. Download an app that filters out blue light.

8. Use an orange gel filter over your screen or wear amber glasses when you are using a device in the evening or late at night.

• • •

The Gratitude Journal

"If you're worried and you can't sleep, count your blessings instead of sheep."

—IRVING BERLIN

Every evening, Dan gets out his laptop (with its night setting on!) and makes a list of all the good things he experienced that day or the tasks he completed. He writes about anything positive from the day's events and is careful to not add a list of chores still waiting to be done. When he looks at what he has written, he feels a sense of accomplishment and ends the day on a positive note. This little ritual not only gives Dan a way to bring his day to a close and unwind, but it prepares him to drift off to sleep without the weight of the world on his shoulders.

•

Erin has a special notebook she keeps beside her bed. On the cover of the notebook are the words "gratitude journal." Every night before she goes to sleep, she writes about anything she is grateful for. The list of things she captures in the book might feel disconnected for an outsider, but for Erin, she knows the list of things she includes in her journal helps her see and feel good about her day. She may write about visits or phone calls with friends, the enchanting sighting of a bird, an inspiring conversation, a piece of art, or witnessing a beautiful flower or sunset. She fills her journal with positive interactions at work, the kindness of a stranger, her passion for food, her appreciation for her home, or even her thoughts about a great movie. Just like Dan's evening routine, by ending her day with her gratitude journal, Erin gets herself ready to rest by choosing to focus on the positives of her day.

•

A sense of gratitude pulls us out of negative, irritated, or victim-based thinking and makes a significant difference in the overall quality of our lives. It can pull us out of sadness and loneliness. By realizing just how much we have to be grateful for, we can sleep better at night as we drift off with a positive frame of mind.

A gratitude journal is one of the most delightful ways to prepare yourself for a great night of sleep. It is like a soft lullaby that you write yourself. I'm grateful to my friend Martha, who introduced me to this ritual for ending the day. It has many uplifting and relaxing effects.

How can you get started and find out if this approach is right for you? Just before you are ready to go to sleep, grab a piece of paper and write down all the positive occurrences of your day. Even if your day was challenging or tiring, or contained bad news, I am sure you will be able to find something positive to write about. Once you think of one really positive thing, other things will probably come to mind too. You may have had a friendly exchange with a neighbor, a meaningful interaction with someone at work, a special chat with a friend; or you may have traveled somewhere new, enjoyed a few minutes outside taking in nature, read a good book, received a promotion at work, or enjoyed a cup of tea—nothing is too big or too insignificant to note. The good feeling the moment gave you is what matters. Anything you are grateful for can be listed. Once you are ready to climb into bed, it's very likely you will turn off the light and remember the warmth of the day. If trying this approach once made a difference for you, why not consider making it part of a regular routine?

Rather than grabbing a piece of loose paper to document your day, upgrade to a journal that you'll use just for your end-of-the-day ritual. Gratitude journals also come in very handy when you have had a bleak day, as browsing through old entries makes you realize that there is a lot of good in your life.

TIPS TO CONSIDER WHEN STARTING
A GRATITUDE JOURNAL

1. **Choose a journal, notepad, diary, or composition book.** Even a piece of loose paper will work fine, but for the best results, keep all of your completed entries together so that you can reference them over time.

2. **Set a time and place to write every night.** That way, every evening before you start getting ready to sleep, you will develop the habit of making time and space for writing down everything positive and worthwhile you remember from your day. Fill the pages of your gratitude journal with all the kindness you experienced during the day, or beauty you witnessed or received. Positive interactions or circumstances of any kind can be written down— everything uplifting and worthwhile you can

remember. Any small event, people you interacted with, beauty you observed, or sweetness you encountered. Write (or even draw) in your book to your heart's content!

3. **Consider keeping a second book for "unloading."** Once you've established the habit of writing in a journal, you might find yourself wanting to write more about your day. If that's the case, remember to manage the purpose behind the action. Keep a second book if you care to journal or process events, interactions, or situations that are more challenging. Processing through journaling is a wonderful way to understand yourself better and let go of life's challenges or emotions.

4. **End your day on the positive.** If you do begin to let go of what's bothering you in a separate journal, make sure you end the evening with your gratitude journal. The warm feelings stirred by keeping a gratitude journal will linger long after you close your journal, and help you get to sleep.

5. **Keep your journal close to your bed.** By having your journal in a place that's easy to find on your side of the bed, you will always be able to access it

quickly for future use and reference, which fosters the daily routine. It is a good idea to start your entry when you still feel awake and alert. Pushing it too close to your self-prescribed bedtime may result in feeling too sleepy to write anything.

• • •

Part II:

**Techniques for
Soothing Insomnia**

EVEN IF YOU HAVE ESTABLISHED a healthy sleep routine, you may still experience sleeplessness from time to time. There are many different causes of insomnia; there are just as many solutions and tools to call on to help you get your z's. In this part of the book, we will explore sixteen techniques for soothing insomnia.

• • •

TECHNIQUE 5

The Eyebrow Sleep Point

Acupressure is a very powerful balancing tool and can be especially helpful as a modality to help encourage better sleep. Acupressure point stimulation assists the body, mind, and consciousness simultaneously. When a person is treated with acupuncture or acupressure, the practitioner may have a certain strategy or approach to healing in mind and choose acupressure points accordingly. It is important to keep in mind that our bodies have a very smart self-healing mechanism. I like to tell my clients that our bodies and minds choose the level of healing they want to receive. Modern medicine tells us that our bodies and minds are well connected. Since they work together very closely, constantly monitoring and influencing one another, many practitioners of both traditional and natural medicine consider them to be one unit, the "body-mind." Consequently, when we receive the healing stimulation of acupressure, it benefits us on all levels: our body relaxes, our mind is able to let go of emotions, and our consciousness becomes more open and balanced.

There is an acupressure point known to acupuncturists as "UB 2" (not to get too technical, but it stands for "urinary bladder meridian point number two") that has been known to deeply relax people and induce sleep. I remember being in an acupuncture class where our teacher wanted to demonstrate the proper needling technique of point UB 2. After having had a few nights of poor sleep, I was eager to be the guinea pig in front of the class. The results were fantastic! After about ten minutes, I couldn't keep my eyes open! I needed to excuse myself from class and go take a nap.

HOW TO DO IT

1. Using both of your thumbs or index fingers, locate the inner-most part of your eyebrows.

2. Pressing the skin right beside the root of your nose, you can feel the upper edge of your eye socket under your fingers. Gently move your fingertips right and left, and you may feel a small notch indicating that you are in the correct spot.

3. With your fingertips properly positioned, apply firm pressure directly onto this area or make small circles over this point with your fingertips. It may feel tender or sore, indicating that your body will be glad to receive a massage in that spot. Tenderness over an acupressure point usually means that this point requires balancing, so you'll know you are doing something your body needs. Again, your body will tell you what you require in order to be healthy. Please listen to yourself!

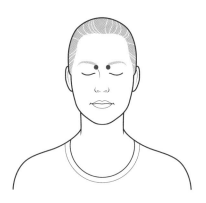

Stimulating this point is known to induce sleep by relaxing the body-mind and the ever-working brain.

4. Apply enough pressure to elicit the desired stimulation and the feeling that is right for you, but not enough to produce pain.

. . .

TECHNIQUE 6

Peaceful Z's

The healing modality of acupressure is a very powerful way of balancing the body and stimulating the body's own self-healing mechanisms. While most acupressure points are on prescribed pathways, known as the "acupuncture channels," the acupressure point known as "Anmian" lies outside these pathways. It is referred to as an "extra point," and it is a wonderful point to help with insomnia. Translated for our understanding, the name Anmian means "peaceful sleep," a promise it has fulfilled for many people.

Insomnia is never easy to contend with, but Anmian can show us a new way. In traditional Chinese medicine, it is believed that the Anmian point anchors both the spirit and mind, so treating this point is indicated for insomnia, agitated and interrupted sleep, and also excessive dreaming.

•

HOW TO DO IT

The sleep point known as Anmian is located on the side of your neck, in the vicinity of your earlobe. It is found halfway between the depression behind your earlobe and the center of your neck (the spot where your head ends and your spine begins).

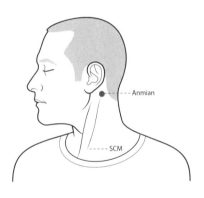

It is beneficial to take slow and full breaths while applying this technique.

1. Place your fingers behind either of your ear-lobes. Using your fingertips, travel backward in a straight line, toward the back of your neck. You will end up moving your fingers approximately one to one and a half inches. Your fingers will travel over the top of a muscle that extends down the side of your neck, the muscle commonly called the "SCM." Once your fingertips have traveled over the muscle, they will find a hollow spot. That is the Anmian acupressure point.

2. Apply pressure to this spot with your thumb or index finger. Move your finger in a small circular motion to increase the effectiveness of balancing this point. In moving your finger in a circular fashion, you may start to feel the base of your skull at certain angles. This anatomical feature will help you know that you are in the correct spot.

3. Massage the Anmian area for two to five minutes or until you instinctively feel you are done.

4. Then, start on the other side of your neck. Once you have gotten used to it, you might be able to massage both sides at the same time.

Most people find that massaging the Anmian area feels relaxing. Do this technique as often as you need to, to promote better sleep and well-being.

• • •

TECHNIQUE 7

Mind Your Heel

My client Jeff had a difficult time falling asleep on and off throughout his life. It wasn't until he learned about the acupressure point on our heels that encourages sleep that he found real results. Once Jeff tried out this technique at bedtime, he was very excited to report that a bit of pressure on his heel as he started winding down for the day had a great result—he soon found himself falling asleep more easily.

The heel point that supports good sleep is another example of an "extra point" in acupressure. While this point lies outside of the regular pathway system used to map acupressure points, it has been proven to be very effective. Because of its ability to deliver on its promises for a sound night's sleep, it has been incorporated into the larger, accepted acupressure system.

The point on your foot to help you sleep is quite easy to find because it is located at the very center of the sole of your heel.

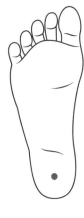

Massage this point just before bedtime or any time you are struggling to get to sleep.

1. Start out by taking a few slow, deep breaths; continue breathing deeply and be mindful of your breathing throughout this exercise.

2. Find the center of your heel, and start to stimulate this point with your thumb. Repeatedly push your thumb right into the center of your heel. Apply deep pressure for about five to ten seconds, and repeat this up to ten times.

3. You may want to use small circular motions to further stimulate this point.

4. Repeat the same process on your other foot.

Should you have trouble reaching your heel, you may want to try using a tool, such as the eraser end of a pencil. You can also gently massage this point by putting a marble or small ball on the floor and gently stepping on it or rolling over it with the center of your heel. Create *just enough* pressure to feel good, but stop short of creating any feelings of pain. As always, listen to your body.

• • •

TECHNIQUE 8

Soothe Your Achy Heart

By the time she came to see me, Clare had not been sleeping well for a year. Every night, she felt tired enough to go to sleep, but as soon as she went to bed and *tried* to go to sleep, she would just lie there, tossing and turning, but not drifting off into dreamland.

In the year before her insomnia set in, Clare had lost her beloved horse. She had had a difficult time dealing with the loss. The years of working with her horse had created a tight bond between them, and while she felt she had gone through her grieving process, she had not entirely let go. The truth was that her grief had gone "underground"; seemingly gone from the surface, it was still present underneath. Helping her let go of her old sadness enabled her to sleep much more soundly.

•

Grief is a known cause of insomnia. We may be aware of our grief and sense of loss, or we may have pushed the emotion away after some time, unaware that our sense of loss is disrupting our sleep. Whether your grief or sense of missing someone or something is old or recent, this technique using specific acupressure points can shift your well-being and heal your tender heart for better sleep. A more sound sleep helps us process, cope, and feel better.

HOW TO DO IT

1. Start by looking at your palm.

2. Place the thumb of your opposite hand at the base of your little finger, and then slide your thumb down the side of your palm toward your wrist. Right after clearing the elevation where your hand ends and your wrist begins, your thumb will settle into a soft depression that rests at the outside edge of your inner wrist. This acupressure point is known to acupuncturists as "Heart 7." This is the point on your wrist that can help address how grief may be affecting your sleep.

3. The second acupressure point for mending your heart is known as "Pericardium 6." To find it, look at your palm once again.

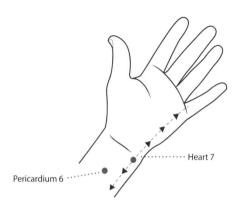

Pericardium 6 ·········· Heart 7

4. Put your index finger of your opposite hand on the center of the crease of your wrist, right by the very end of your palm; then move your finger approximately 2.5 to 3 inches down toward the lower portion of your wrist. The point for which you are searching is in the very center of your forearm, just up from your wrist. If you are having trouble finding Pericardium 6, then place three of your fingers—your ring, middle, and index fingers—on your wrist crease, just under your palm. The pressure point Pericardium 6 will be located just under your index finger, in the center of your forearm.

5. Once you find these points on your arm, apply strong but comfortable pressure with your thumb or any other finger for about a minute or so—first to one point, then the other.

6. Then, repeat on your other wrist.

There's no harm in repeating this process several times. As with other techniques, listen to your body. Apply the pressure that feels right for you, for however long feels right for you.

• • •

TECHNIQUE 9

Calm and Sleepy

We usually think that insomnia has much to do with our heads, our minds. *If only our brain could settle down so we could drift off to restful sleep!* While the ankle seems a long way from the head, the acupressure points recommended in this technique have been proven to correct our sleeping patterns and resolve insomnia. There are acupressure meridians on either side of the ankle that actually connect to the head. Massaging the points on this meridian helps balance the brain and our thoughts. These two acupressure points, which are just below your ankles on both sides of your feet, are "sleep points" known to have worked wonders for many people with insomnia.

·

HOW TO DO IT

1. Start by giving yourself a good stretch by raising your arms and lifting them toward the sky. Feel how your muscles and joints enjoy this movement. A few gentle sideways movements will open your torso as well. Take a few deep breaths; if you can, you may want to try to induce or indulge in a good yawn as well.

2. Sitting in a comfortable chair with your legs just a few inches apart, bring your right lower leg to rest on top of your left thigh. If your body is feeling very tight, and it is difficult for you to rest your lower leg on your opposite thigh, try putting your right foot on a low table or chair in front of you.

3. Put your thumb on one side of your ankle and your index finger on the other side. If you have small hands, or have a difficult time stretching your hands across your ankles, know that you can massage these points separately if it is easier for you. The acupressure point known as "K 6" is located on the inside of your ankle, in a little hollow that sits about one inch below your

anklebone. On the outside of your ankle, about half an inch below the anklebone, rests the acupressure point "UB 62."

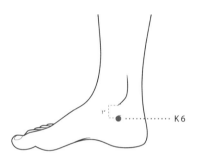

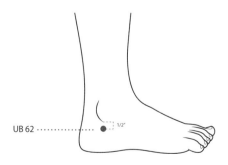

4. Once you've located these spots, use your thumb and index finger—or whatever finger feels most comfortable to you—and give the acupressure points a massage by making very small, mindful circles with your fingertips.

5. Massage the points for about four minutes, taking slow, deep breaths while you are doing so. If you are able, end the process by inducing another yawn, just to get your body embracing the need for sleep.

6. Repeat the same process on the other foot. For best results, massage these acupressure points a few times during the day and then again before bedtime.

• • •

TECHNIQUE 10

Circle Your Ear

Ear acupuncture is not just self-help; it is a powerful healing modality I focused on quite a bit in the other 5-Minute First Aid for the Mind books, which cover reducing cravings and relieving stress. The ear is considered one of the "reflex organs." Each part of the body, as well as each emotional state, has an area of representation on the ear. As a result, acupuncture or acupressure performed on the ear can assist in balancing the corresponding parts of the body.

Usually, when there is an imbalance in the body-mind, the corresponding ear acupressure point feels somewhat tender. In addition, it is more "electrically active," meaning that the center of the acupressure point has lowered electrical resistance in contrast to the surrounding skin. This can easily be verified with an ohmmeter, a device that measures electrical resistance. Our bodies are indeed wondrous!

While we won't be further exploring ohmmeters and electrical resistance, it's important to understand the intricacies of energy captured in your ear and how they can be used to get a better night's sleep. This approach to "auriculotherapy" (literally, "ear therapy") gets your body-mind to a state of relaxation, enabling you to fall and stay asleep.

HOW TO DO IT

Take a few deep and slow breaths. Feel the rise and fall of both your belly and chest as you breathe. Close your eyes if that feels right to you.

1. Take one of your fingers—I suggest your index or middle finger—and slowly circle the outside circumference of your ear with either the tip or side of your finger. Start right on the small, soft flap of cartilage that protects your ear canal, which is called the "tragus."

2. From that flap, move your finger up to the top of your ear, then along the outer edge of your ear, down and around to your earlobe. From the bottom lobe of your ear, move gently back up to your ear's tragus.

3. Repeat this motion slowly as you also try to slow down your cycle of breath. As you circle your ear, you may want to stop around your earlobe; placing your thumb and index finger on either side of your earlobe, give it a flat, mindful pinch.

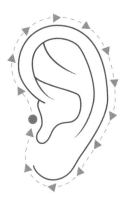

By moving your finger along the outer edge of your ear, you slow down your nervous system. Calming the system that drives your body's get-up-and-go impulses, you may feel a gentle calming feeling take over your body. The earlobe contains many corresponding points for the face, brain, and emotions. If you lightly pinch or touch the earlobes as if rubbing two sides of a coin between your fingertips, you can help balance tensions across various areas of your body, which prepares you to float off to sleep.

• • •

TECHNIQUE 11

Pinch Your Toes

We take much in life for granted. For instance, we walk on our feet all day long without any concern for the magnificent task with which they are presented—carrying us around. Unless we have a splinter, an injury, or a sharp object that immediately redirects our attention to our feet, we tend not to focus on them at all. Our feet have many more good qualities about them. They do more for us than simply provide transportation.

The science of "reflexology" tells us the soles of our feet can help heal any part of our body. Receiving a foot massage, or foot reflexology, can be very relaxing. It allows us to be more present in our bodies, which in turn helps us sleep better; by resting and sleeping we can stimulate our bodies' innate healing response.

When preoccupied with work or other issues in our lives, we seem to be in a different world. We are inhabiting a space outside of our bodies. Foot reflexology is a technique that can reconnect our minds with our bodies, giving us more presence of mind. As Eckhart Tolle assures us in his book *The Power of Now,* "All power lies in the present moment." Truly resting and being able to sleep well greatly enhances our ability to focus and live in the present.

Here's where your feet come in to all of this. The webs of your toes carry many nerve fibers that connect to your nervous system. While we are going about our day focused on tasks, we are primarily under the influence of one part of the nervous system, called the sympathetic nervous system. The sympathetic nervous system gives us our get-up-and-go response. However, in the evening we rely on a completely different part of the nervous system to help us relax and rejuvenate—the parasympathetic nervous system. The parasympathetic system helps us find balance, relaxing and restoring us. This system helps us drift off to sleep and allows our bodies' immune and healing systems to kick in to get us ready for the next day.

Stimulating the web between your toes helps you relax and switch from the get-up-and-go of the sympathetic nervous system to the heal-and-relax mode of the parasympathetic nervous system. Massaging while squeezing the top and bottom of the webbing between your toes is akin to pushing the reset button on your nervous system or telling your computer to shut down at the end of the day. This technique helps take a body that may be stuck in activity mode into settle-down mode.

HOW TO DO IT

Take off your shoes and socks and start with bare feet. Find a comfortable position.

1. Rest one of your feet on your opposite thigh or on a chair in front of you.

2. Take a few deep breaths and massage the sole of your foot.

3. Apply a mindful amount of pressure to your foot with your thumbs, concentrating on the areas that feel tender or in need of attention. While there is no need to use any lotion or oil during this process, feel free to do so if you like. Pay special attention to your toes. If it is comfortable for you, web your fingers between your toes and move your toes in all directions.

4. Stretch your toes apart, spreading them as much as you can. Rest your thumb on the top and your index finger on the bottom part of the web between two of your toes. Even if you cannot spread your toes very far, you can still get a hold of the web.

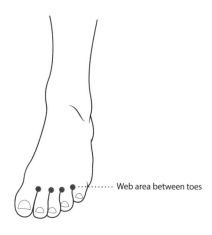

Web area between toes

5. Give this area a firm, slow squeeze, but be mindful not to rub or massage the area too much. Press on this area for five to ten seconds and then quickly release it.

Can you feel the effect this release has in your body-mind? Repeat the "web-squeeze" between each of your toes, across both of your feet. As always, listen to your own body regarding the amount of pressure you apply and be mindful of your breath throughout this technique. Be sure to take slow, deep breaths.

• • •

TECHNIQUE 12

The Fountain of Sleep

Our foreheads reveal much about our state of being. Pronounced lines across the forehead may show deep thought and worry. A raised eyebrow or two show surprise or disbelief. A smooth forehead indicates relaxation and ease of mind.

As an acupuncturist, I have, time and again, noticed the profound relaxation brought about by the needling of a point called "yintang," which is located between the eyebrows. Oftentimes, clients' thoughts are much more at ease after a treatment that includes the yintang point, and some even say they notice a feeling of relaxation across their forehead muscles lasting for many hours. Along with the relaxation of the muscles of the forehead comes a relaxation of the mind. Coincidentally or not, the forehead covers our frontal brain, our center of thinking, which houses our powers of reasoning and ruminating. After you make that connection, perhaps it's easy to see how acupressure techniques centering on the yintang point can help you relax, let go of your day, and prepare for a sound night of z's.

HOW TO DO IT

1. Using your index or middle fingers, place one finger from each hand between your eyebrows so that they are just above the root of your nose.

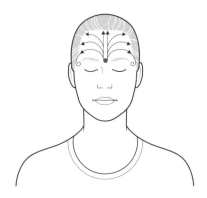

2. Starting from the point just between your eyebrows, guide your fingers upward and outward in a slow and repetitive movement.

3. Breathe in and out slowly and deeply. This is another example of how listening to your body and your needs can help your relaxation. Use the degree of pressure that feels right for you at the time. Some days you might need just a gentle touch. Other days you may want to apply more pressure across your forehead to get the desired result.

4. As you move upward and outward, imagine you are tracing the movements of a fountain that flows water in the shape of a palm tree. When you move your fingers toward your temples, you may want to massage your temple muscles with a few circular motions. Pay special attention to any small knots in the underlying muscles of your temples. A little massage will help soften them—and your emotions.

Keep breathing slowly and notice the wonderful calming effect of this technique. You may notice that your thoughts calm down and your forehead feels more relaxed and less crunched from overthinking.

As we ruminate over our daily stresses, we unconsciously tighten. As we prepare for sleep, we have to create the time and opportunity to release these tensions we carry in our bodies. This exercise gives us the routine with which to do that, and has the added benefit of softening our thoughts and smoothing our frowns and wrinkles.

• • •

The Sleep Mantra

Maria is a very busy woman. She has a big family and faces many challenges in her professional and personal life. When she came for a consultation during a particularly stressful time in her life, I expected her sleep to be disrupted. To my surprise, she did not come to me for help with her sleep. *I* learned a lesson about sleep *from her.* Upon my inquiring about her sleep patterns, she said: "I actually sleep just fine. When my thoughts are too busy, I say the sleep mantra. I repeat the word 'sleep' very slowly, again and again, until I drift off. Usually it does not take long to feel the relaxation setting in, and I feel my head sinking into the pillow more and more."

•

Miguel builds beautiful homes and is an avid musician. When Miguel has trouble falling asleep, he slowly recites the lyrics to his favorite songs. He says, "Most of the time, I fall asleep while reciting the first song or two. If I am still wide awake after reciting the lyrics to three songs, I usually read for a little while until I feel more tired. Taking slow, deep breaths while remembering the lyrics always helps me as well."

•

I had a lot to learn from both Maria's and Miguel's techniques. This was confirmed when yet another client, named Sabina, told me that on the nights her thoughts swirl around and around in her head preventing her from sleeping, she relies on a mantra to re-center herself. She recites the words "calm, calm, calm . . ." over and over again in her mind to help clear her thoughts. She told me, "If you really concentrate on the word 'calm,' your mind cannot think about all those swirling thoughts at the same time. It always helps me fall asleep."

•

A mantra is a word or short sentence that is usually repeated slowly and purposefully, allowing your mind to reach deeper levels of concentration. Initially designed as a focusing tool for meditation, a mantra helps you let go of the chatter in your mind. It can be repeated silently and mindfully, or aloud.

While the word "mantra" stems from Buddhism and Hinduism, you can use any word or sentence in any language as a mantra. It is, however, important to make it a positive and relevant statement. Some people prefer a mantra in a different language, as it helps disengage their minds from thinking too much about the meaning.

Borrowing the mantra technique to fall asleep has been helpful for many people. As a matter of fact, when my friends heard that I was collecting techniques to help people improve their quality of sleep, many approached me wanting to share this technique, as they found it to be a most useful tool. Just like Maria, use a simple word or a phrase that helps you calm down your thoughts and relax into sleep.

HOW TO DO IT

On those nights you find yourself unable to fall asleep, take a few deep breaths in and out. Focus your attention on the feeling of the pillow under your head and neck, the mattress supporting you, and the sheets covering you.

Close your eyes and think of a positive or neutral word or phrase that is soothing or helps distract you from revolving thoughts. Keep repeating it slowly and mindfully. This keeps your mind from being preoccupied with seemingly pressing ideas, tasks, or emotions. As you repeat your mantra, pay attention to your body. Zero in on any stress in your body, and let go of any muscle tension, one muscle at a time, every time your exhale. As you do, relax into the soft embrace of your bed.

Use any mantra that comes to your mind. Here are a few examples from which you can choose:

- *Sleep, sleep, sleep . . .*

- [As you inhale] *I relax.*
  [As you exhale] *I feel my muscles let go.*

- [As you inhale] *Who am I?*
  [As you exhale] *I don't know.*

- Count your breaths; when you have counted to five, start over again.

- *Calm, calm, calm . . .*

- *Om Mani Padme Hum.* This is a famous Sanskrit mantra that is thought to contain all of the teachings of the Buddha in its sound. It is used as a calming tool for meditation and will most likely benefit your sleep as well. This mantra's words translate to mean wisdom (*om*), compassionate mind (*mani*), equanimity and bliss (*padme*), and quality of compassion (*hum*).

TECHNIQUE 14

Brown Bag Sleep

Kiaan has a very busy job overseeing city planning. His day is full of many meetings, deadlines, and never-ending correspondence. At times, when attempting to go to sleep at night, his mind goes over the numerous communications he exchanged during the day, or the phone calls and e-mails still to be completed.

In the practice of meditation, there is a term to represent this seemingly aimless drifting of thoughts we experience. When your mind jumps from one thing to another, it is called "monkey-mind." Calming the monkey-mind helps you focus your mind for meditation, and it can do the same as you fall asleep.

In working with Kiaan, we found a visualization technique that has been very helpful in allowing his mind to take a break from the constant chatter of monkey-mind. He reimagines the tasks he still needs to complete, or the fragments of conversation running through his mind, as tennis balls. As the thoughts come to his awareness, he imagines he is playing a game of tennis. As thoughts form, they are transformed into tennis balls and he is able to hit them back over the net and away from him. Playing tennis with his thoughts gives his mind a focus of a different kind.

•

Many times when Julie tries to fall asleep, no matter how tired she is, thoughts about her day come flooding in. Julie, like many of us, is processing the events of her day as she begins to settle in for the night. Snippets of information drift into her awareness, and she thinks of tasks that need to be done or how she can improve things that were already completed. Sometimes it is just emotions that take over her mind. On nights like that, Julie loves a technique that she learned in a class: the brown paper bag technique. She imagines a brown paper bag right beside her bed; when thoughts come into her mind, she thanks them for appearing and imagines putting them into the brown paper bag. "It really helps me let go of my thoughts. Of course, as soon as I put one thought into the bag, the next one appears, so I have to keep doing it until my mind calms down. Then all I remember is waking up the next morning."

•

Whether you imagine your thoughts or feelings as tennis balls that you can hit across a court or imagine a bag into which you pour the contents of your day, the techniques shared by Kiaan and Julie can be used to your benefit as you approach the end of your day and crave some restful sleep.

HOW TO DO IT

When your mind is distracted with thoughts, tasks, or emotions, take a few deep breaths. Imagine a large, sturdy, brown paper bag right beside your bed, open and ready to receive the contents floating around your mind that are distracting you from sleep.

As those distractions surface in your mind, give thanks to them for reminding you of their presence. They occur for a good reason after all, and you may want to pay attention to them at a time when you are more rested. But at that moment, imagine wiping your hand across your forehead, picking up the thought or emotion, and dropping it into the brown paper bag right beside you. Your imaginary paper bag is bottomless, much like Mary Poppins's magical bag. Within it, there is plenty of space, and it can contain everything you toss in it, keeping things safe for later use or processing.

If the symbol of the bag doesn't calm you as much, and you find something like Kiaan's tennis balls more appealing, then follow that format. Hockey pucks, footballs, badminton birdies, or something else could easily be swapped in, if you find it more appealing. Visualize your thoughts as a form that is easy for you to toss aside. Whatever helps you let them go is what you should follow.

• • •

TECHNIQUE 15

Betty Erickson's Sleep Induction

For Jackson, bedtime comes with a set of expected scenarios. As he says, "When I go to bed at night, something predictable happens. I am glad to go to bed; I am tired and look forward to a good sleep. I snuggle into my nice and welcoming bed, and then my mind takes me on a journey far away. I revisit conversations I had during the previous day or two or years ago, I make phone calls in my mind, revisit perceived slights against me, and solve problems that require a solution—but not right at that very moment!"

During nights like those, Jackson says the Betty Erickson technique of sleep induction is his favorite technique to call on. Betty's technique helps people return mentally, emotionally, and physically to where they are at that moment—their comfortable bed—and helps them relax and realize it's time to drift off to sleep.

Our minds are very powerful and create the reality in which we find ourselves. In our minds, we live either in harmony or anger or fear. We adhere to conversations, emotions, opinions, and relationship dynamics, whether or not it serves our mental and physical health. Negative thoughts have a strong effect on how our bodies function and have been shown to wind down our immune system, reduce our energy level, tighten our muscles, make us more accident-prone, and diminish our sense of well-being.

When your mind cannot settle down or focus on one thing, it is even easier to dwell on the challenges you have encountered. You might find yourself returning time and time again to what is *not* going well in your life, particularly at the end of the day when you should be drifting off to sleep. As I mentioned in Technique 14, there is a term in the practice of meditation to represent this seemingly aimless drifting of thoughts we experience—it is called "monkey-mind." With monkey-mind, we are led on a playful journey to wherever our minds want us to go. Fortunately, there are tried and tested techniques that can bring us back into our bodies at the present moment, ground us in the reality of the here and now, and allow us to listen to what our bodies need. We know that all power lies in the present moment—especially when we are in the process of going to sleep.

This sleep induction technique was developed by Betty Erickson, the wife of psychiatrist, hypnosis therapist, and lecturer Dr. Milton Erickson. It is a beautiful technique because of its simplicity. It is effective and taps into the power of our minds. Betty's technique is a version of self-hypnosis that tames the monkey-mind and promotes better sleep.

HOW TO DO IT

1. Begin by making yourself comfortable.

2. Find something within the room that you can *see* around you to focus on. For example, one corner of a door frame, a light switch, or a cherished object. Then, maintaining your focus on that one item, try to notice four specific things about that item or spot in the room. For example:

   • What color is it?
   • Does it have texture?

- Is it shiny or flat in appearance?
- What shape is it?

3. Look for and focus on details that you had not noticed before, and mentally feed them back to yourself. For the greatest benefit, use the phrase "Right now, I can see . . ." to mentally message what you see back to yourself. Add the details of the object on which you are focused. For example:
   - Right now, I can see the light switch is white.
   - Right now, I can see the shadow at the edge of the switch.
   - Right now, I can see the switch is a square shape.
   - Right now, I can see the switch is in the off position.

4. This example list has four things. This simple list of four things helps you focus on what you see around you.

5. Next, try to notice all the things you can *hear*. Using the same type of script, make four statements to yourself about what you hear.

For example:

- Right now, I hear the sound of the air conditioner.
- Right now, I hear the sound of the clock ticking.
- Right now, I hear voices in the next room.
- Right now, I hear cars passing by outside.

6. Again, by using the phrase "Right now, I hear…" before each item, we are brought back to the here and now with a simple list of four things.

7. The next step is to notice all the things you can physically *feel*. Using a similar script as before, begin to list to yourself one sensation at a time. For example:

- Right now, I feel the sheets covering me.
- Right now, I feel the softness of the mattress below me.
- Right now, I feel the pillow under my head.
- Right now, I feel the soft fabric of my pajamas.

8. Having listed three sets of things you notice — what you see, hear, and feel—start the process

over again. Look for new things that you see, but this time list *three* qualities of an object instead of four.

9. After listing the three qualities of the new item you see, list three new things that you hear, and three new things you feel.

10. Repeat the process again, but list only *two* things you see, hear, and feel.

11. Finally, repeat the process again, listing only *one* thing in each category.

It's worth noting that you will probably run out of different things to hear or feel. In these cases, it's fine to repeat something you noticed earlier. But do try to find different things. You may be surprised at how much more you can notice that doesn't seem obvious at first.

• • •

TECHNIQUE 16

Liver Time List

"I am an insomniac; my mind works the night shift."
—PETE WENTZ

Insomnia presents with various patterns. Understanding the differences among the patterns will be an important step in alleviating your sleep issues.

"Initial insomnia" refers to the inability to fall asleep when first closing our eyes to go to sleep. Another variety, "duration insomnia," means that we have no problems falling asleep, but wake up during the night only to find ourselves too awake to drift back off.

Traditional Chinese medicine (TCM), with its three-thousand-year history, can give us a deeper appreciation of the internal dynamics of our sleep patterns. The principles of TCM can help us find the underlying causes and patterns of our sleep problems, which can help tremendously with finding a solution to our dilemma. One of the most useful concepts in

TCM is the "Chinese organ clock," which gives us clues we can use to help ourselves experience a restful night. The Chinese organ clock, or Chinese meridian clock, follows the understanding that our life energy courses through a series of energy channels ("meridians") within our bodies, and that this energy pulses at a steady rhythm. Our body energy, also known as "Chi," moves along a prescribed path throughout the day and night. It spends two hours of "focused energy" in each meridian. That means it is paying extra attention to certain organs at the same two-hour time interval throughout the course of the entire day, every day. To explore the Chinese organ clock on your own and gain a deeper understanding behind its concepts, please see part 4 of this book.

According to the Chinese organ clock, between the hours of 1 a.m. and 3 a.m., your energy is focused at your liver meridian. So, people who experience duration insomnia between the hours of 1 a.m. and 3 a.m. may have an imbalance of their liver energy. This does not mean that your liver is "sick," however; it means that the energy of your liver needs support. We know that the liver is responsible for digesting our food and detoxifying our bodies. It should come as no surprise if we find ourselves wide awake around "liver time" after consuming a heavy meal or too much alcohol. However, TCM can help us understand that the liver meridian is also responsible for supporting the planning and organizing functions in our minds. Some of us may find that our minds are very active around "liver time," and that it is within this time frame that we suddenly gain a great sense of clarity. At the best of times, we may suddenly awake knowing the perfect wording for an e-mail or letter we need to write, a presentation we are to give, or any other creative endeavor. At other times, our liver energy may wake us up so that we may go through lists of chores to be completed, reminding ourselves at this inopportune time of phone calls we need to make or tasks that need to be completed. Having spent a good amount of time planning and organizing, we might finally fall asleep again, only to have the morning alarm lift us out of a dream state when we least want it.

If you regularly wake up between 1 and 3 a.m., and you know that heavy food and drink isn't the main trigger for your liver-time wake-up call, then your goal is to learn to work with your liver channel's support for your mind. Learning to anticipate the organization and planning your liver and mind might do in the wee hours of the morning is a technique that will help you relax and fall back asleep more quickly.

HOW TO DO IT

Keep a notepad or journal and a pen beside your bed. If you've read Technique 4 and have chosen to adopt the ritual of keeping a gratitude journal, make sure that you use a different journal for this purpose. Journals used as tools, such as these, should help you focus on specific things. Your focus on gratitude should be kept separate from your problem solving, and hence it requires a separate journal.

When you wake to find yourself flooded with brilliant ideas, stories, or insights, write them down in your journal for safekeeping. Immediately set the habit of getting the thoughts out and into your journal so that they don't sit in your mind, where you will continue to dwell on them. This process will become a routine that will have two beneficial effects. First, you will have a tool that will help remind you of the often clear and eloquent thoughts you had in the middle of the night. After waking from interrupted sleep, it is hard to face the morning and remember the insights that might have woken you in the first place. Second, the process will unburden your mind and prevent any ideas from taking up space in your memory bank the next day. You may find yourself drifting off to sleep much faster knowing that the pressing issues and brilliant solutions have been recorded and will be ready for you to tackle at a more appropriate time.

• • •

TECHNIQUE 17

Get Up and Try Again

"If at first you don't succeed, get up and try again."
—ANONYMOUS

At times, we retire to bed looking forward to a good night's sleep only to find that our mind wakes up and becomes perky once we hit the pillow. At other times, we fall asleep just fine only to suddenly wake from a deep sleep in the middle of the night, our mind suddenly busy with seemingly pressing tasks like folding the laundry, sorting papers, making phone calls, or sending urgent e-mails. It is on nights like these, when your mind will not quiet down, that we might need to remind ourselves of the old adage that there is always room to try again.

If you try some of the relaxation exercises in this book, but still cannot get to sleep, you may want to just get up and engage in some activity. On nights like that, know you are not alone. The wisdom keepers of sound sleep have experienced this problem and are the first to admit that there are times when getting out of bed and moving might actually be exactly what you need for a good night of sleep. Get up and try again, by tackling mundane and boring tasks that do not require a lot of brain function and mental alertness. You'll end up with a sense of accomplishment, and you will have moved your body a little, which often helps settle a person back into dreamland.

HOW TO DO IT

If you find yourself too alert to get to sleep and feel that your body would rather engage in activity, get out of bed and tackle a small and mundane task for fifteen minutes or so. The short burst of physical activity will reset your nervous system. Then, when you are done, go back to bed. You may notice that your body wanted a little movement and productivity before settling down for the night.

Here are some sample sleep-enhancing tasks to do at night:

- Arrange your dishes
- Mend a sock
- Sort your recycling (if it does not wake your housemates)

- Make lunches for the next day

- Fold laundry

- Clean out your purse

- Trim your moustache

- Alphabetize your book shelf

- Dust your trophies

- Read a ho-hum book

When getting up at night, it is important to remember to stay away from electronic screens of any kind. It is wise to avoid cell phones, computers, tablets, e-readers, or video games, as such activities may rouse your nervous system rather than settle it down. Should there be an urgent need to use an electronic device, make sure the night setting is turned on to protect your body from the blue and white hues that signal daytime to your nervous system.

• • •

TECHNIQUE 18

Breathe Yourself to Sleep

Our next technique, alternate nostril breathing, is a tried and true tool inspired by the world of yoga. Even if you're not a yoga practitioner, you can use alternate nostril breathing to manage stress and insomnia.

Like many other breathing exercises, you will find that alternating your breath between your nostrils helps calm your nervous system. The process grounds your thoughts, enabling you to fall asleep more easily. I do this technique quite regularly, and yet I never cease to be astonished by how easily and quickly I feel it soften my body, mind, and spirit.

At first, the process seems a little complex. But know that it becomes very easy after you practice it a few times. The goal is to bring a sense of calm and mindfulness to your breathing, which in turn balances the relaxation part of your nervous system.

HOW TO DO IT

1. Hold your right hand up in front of you and look at your palm.

2. Bend your index and middle fingers. Your hand will look like this:

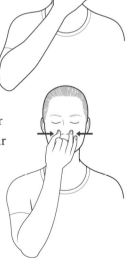

3. Place your thumb over your right nostril to restrict the airflow into your right nostril and slowly breathe in to the count of four through your left nostril.

4. Use your ring finger to cover your left nostril. Both of your nostrils are now blocked, allowing you to hold your breath. Hold your breath for a count of four.

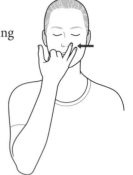

5. Release your thumb, allowing yourself to deeply exhale through your right nostril.

6. Start over, breathing in through your right nostril for a count of four.

7. Hold your breath for a count of four while closing both nostrils and then release your ring finger and exhale through your left nostril for a count of four.

8. Keep breathing like this for three minutes or so, and finish by exhaling on the left side (starting and finishing breathing on the left side completes full rounds of breathing).

9. Relax into your being while continuing to breathe slowly. You may feel a deepened sense of tranquility, allowing you to fall asleep.

• • •

TECHNIQUE 19

6, 7, 8, Sleep!

When it comes to tools that help in catching some z's, there are few things as miraculous as slowing down your breath. Slow and deliberate breathing not only gives your body and brain much-needed oxygen, but also shifts your nervous system to the heal-and-relax phase, which is supported by the parasympathetic nervous system. Slow, deep breathing helps induce sleep by relaxing your muscles and your thoughts. You may find that it acts like a natural tranquilizer, which can also make it a go-to tool to use at any time of the day or night when you might find yourself needing a little calm.

The key to this technique is to achieve balance between the inhalation and exhalation rhythm in your breathing. That is, when you breathe in for almost the same amount of time that you breathe out, your overall pattern of breathing is slowed down. When your breath is slowed down, your body-mind slows down.

The process is most helpful when you shift your focus and awareness to listening to your body's ability to breathe. By listening to your body, and with a little practice, you will achieve a proper ratio between your inhalation and exhalation of air; the more often you use this technique, the easier it will become. Before you know it, you'll be able to call on this technique very quickly to help you unwind.

HOW TO DO IT

Get in a relaxed position. Let go of any tension in your shoulders or jaw. Feel your arms get heavy and your leg muscles soften. Close your eyes and let go of the tension in your eye muscles.

1. With your tongue gently positioned behind your upper teeth, breathe in slowly through your nose to the count of six (or whatever count feels comfortable to you).

2. Hold your breath to the count of seven.

3. Let go of your breath through your mouth to the count of eight. Feel your breath pushing out from your belly and your chest. If possible, keep your tongue resting behind your front teeth for

the entire exercise, as it helps connect important energetic pathways.

4. Keep breathing in this pattern for three to five minutes, or as long as you need to become grounded in calmness.

• • •

TECHNIQUE 20

Unwind Your Spine

As my friend Marco says, "I have been practicing yoga on and off throughout my life. I am not particularly good at it, but whenever I have difficulty sleeping, I go back to doing a few yoga exercises and they always help me relax and feel better."

·

Yoga can be practiced in a very gentle and mindful way. A rigorous approach isn't necessary for results. A soft approach that does not force your body will give you many of the same health benefits. Staying focused on the movement and sensations in our bodies is what grounds us in the here and now. This provides a profound sense of relaxation. In this technique, we'll be focusing on the benefits of yogic stretches for the spine.

HOW TO DO IT

1. Lie down on a flat surface, such as your bed, a carpet, or an exercise mat.

2. Stretch your arms out at your sides so that your body takes a "T" position. With your body flat and relaxed, take a few deep and slow breaths.

3. Rest your right foot on your left knee and allow your bent right knee to fall over to the left side of your body. The position of your leg and the movement in your back will gently twist your spine. If your back is very tense or doesn't have a lot of mobility, know that your knee does not have to move very far to the side for the benefits of this pose—even a few inches will allow this posture to help your body relax. No need to force it!

4. Make sure that your right shoulder maintains contact with the floor, even as your body continues to stretch to the left. Be mindful of how you feel. Be aware of your body and breathe into the sensations you experience.

5. If you can, slowly turn your head to the right and gaze over your right shoulder. Again, only do this if it feels comfortable. If you feel any pain as you attempt to move your neck to the right, then keep your neck centered.

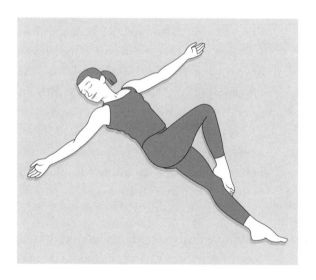

6. Stay in this position for five slow breaths; then move your right knee back up so it points toward the ceiling. Straighten your right leg and lie on your back, enjoying the feeling of unwinding your spine. Take several deep breaths.

7. Follow the same process on the other side of your body.

• • •

Part III:

Techniques for Dealing with Jet Lag

MANY OF US LOVE TO TRAVEL and experience new or favorite destinations. A few hours of flying through the air, and we are able to explore different cultures and climates, take in diverse languages and mentalities, try exotic foods, and admire unfamiliar art and architecture. It is still amazing to me that we load large and heavy planes with luggage, goods, and people and proceed to travel at high altitudes to faraway destinations.

Planning a trip is exciting, and the prospect of spending time in faraway places is enticing; however, time changes and jet lag can interfere with our overall sense of well-being. Minimizing the effects of jet lag enhances our enjoyment of a trip. It can help with mental alertness, make us more mindful (and therefore less prone to injuries), boost our immune system, and enhance our general sense of vitality. Adjusting our bodies and minds to a new time zone gives us that extra sense of wakefulness to enjoy the sights, meet new people, and make the most of our trip.

Managing jet lag is especially important for people who travel for business, because their jobs often require a keen sense of attention shortly after they land. Trips are often taken within very short time frames, to faraway destinations, and time is usually of the essence. If you have a trip in which you will be heading straight to a meeting as soon as you disembark from the plane, or have important business to tackle the morning after your trip, you may benefit greatly from these techniques.

The pieces of advice in this section of the book will show you how to reduce the effects of jet lag. Full of tips commonly shared and applied successfully by many leisure and business travelers, these techniques will help you make the most of your travel time.

• • •

TECHNIQUE 21

Wisdom from the Sages of Jet Lag

1. **Think ahead.** Consider the time change when booking your flight. When traveling east (for example, from North America to Europe), try to book a flight that leaves in the later hours of the evening. This way, you'll be tired when you board the plane. If you are lucky, you will get several hours of sleep as you travel, which will leave you feeling more refreshed when you arrive at your destination in the early morning hours. In contrast, if you leave North America in the early or late afternoon, it might take you several hours to feel tired and finally sleep. By the time you've arrived at your destination, you might have missed an entire night's sleep, making you feel groggy and less able to function for several days at your new location.

2. **Start early.** Here is another example of how planning ahead can go a long way. Before you set off, try to make some adjustments to your regular bedtime. Mirror the time at your destination, and

start adjusting your patterns to match the time zone to which you are traveling. It is more challenging to adjust to a different time zone when traveling east rather than west. The common saying goes, "Traveling west is best, east is a beast." When traveling east, go to sleep and wake earlier than your regular routine; if you are traveling west, stay up later and try to sleep an extra hour or two in the morning.

3. **Reset your watch.** At the start of your trip, change the time on your watch to match the time at your destination.

4. **Drink up!** Make sure you stay well hydrated. Drink as much water as you can!

5. **But avoid alcohol.** It's tempting to indulge and relax as you fly, but remember that alcohol is dehydrating. Your body needs all the water it can get. Alcohol makes time zone adjustments more difficult and only adds to dehydration.

6. **Plan your caffeine.** Remember that it takes four to five hours for caffeine to break down in our bodies. So, avoid that coffee on the plane until you need it. If you need to sleep as you travel and be full of

TECHNIQUE 22

Resetting Your Body Clock

Acclimating your body's inner clock to new sleep and meal times can take many days when traveling across several time zones. This disruption of one's circadian rhythm can result in headaches, mental fogginess, fatigue, memory lapses, and insomnia. I remember traveling to China—a twelve-hour time change from my home—and waking up in the middle of the night for almost a week. My stomach demanded lunch at what was one o'clock in the morning local time.

Acupressure offers a gem of a technique to assist your body and mind as they adjust to your new time zone. Acupressure for jet lag focuses on resetting your inner body and mind clock, known as your "circadian rhythm." Before you know it, this technique may become one of your most useful self-help travel tools.

I have tried this technique many times with great success, and you can start doing it while on the plane to your destination. It usually creates an immediate sense of gentle alertness, and by continuing this technique for a number of days after your arrival, you'll only continue to reap its many benefits.

For this tool, we'll be relying on the "Chinese organ clock," mentioned in Technique 16, which provides us an understanding of each acupressure meridian's specific time of focused activity across the twenty-four hours in each day. Traditional Chinese medicine (TCM) follows the belief that there are twelve meridians in our bodies; energy (or *chi*) flows from one meridian to another in two-hour cycles throughout the day and night. Each meridian has a "focus time" during the course of a day and night when energy in that meridian is enhanced. By following the chart at the end of this technique when you travel and enjoy your destination, you'll work with your body's own energy to reset your circadian rhythms.

HOW TO DO IT

1. Before embarking on your flight, reset your watch to the current time at your destination and visualize yourself being there enjoying the day. Imagine that you are already starting your holiday or getting ready for your business meeting or conference!

2. When settling into your seat on the plane, look up the acupressure point that corresponds to the current time at your destination (see chart that begins on page 121). Apply pressure to the appropriate acupressure point by firmly holding or rubbing that point for approximately two to three minutes. Take some deep, slow breaths in and out while you press on the point. **Repeat the process on the same acupressure point on the other side of your body.** For example, if it is 3 a.m. at the city to which you are traveling, then according to the chart, you will be applying pressure to what acupuncturists refer to as point "Lung 8." The time between 3 and 5 a.m. is "lung time"—meaning that energy is most concentrated in the lung meridian. Your body's natural rhythm will benefit from stimulating that point. You will, therefore, be adjusting your body to the time frames and rhythms of your final destination.

3. According to TCM, the energy within meridians or channels moves every two hours—from one meridian to another. As a result, to make the most of this acupressure technique, it is best

to repeat the process about every two hours. If you are asleep, enjoy your rest; don't feel compelled to wake up and apply the technique. But, do make full use of it during your waking hours. This is important! Only stimulate the acupressure point that is "active" according to the local time at your destination. You will arrive feeling more invigorated and more alert!

4. As you settle in at your destination, continue using this acupressure technique whenever it is convenient for you. It is best to use this technique one day for each hour of time change you accumulated as a result of your trip. For example, for best results, you should rely on this technique for five days if you have crossed five time zones. The more you are able to make use of this tool, the faster your body, mind, and energy will adjust to your new time zone.

Remember: Once you've located the points described in the chart on the next page, repeat the process of applying pressure to the same acupressure point on the other side of your body.

• • •

JET LAG ACUPRESSURE CHART

Time at Destination	Name and Location of Point	How to Find the Point
3–5 a.m.	LUNG 8	Look at the palm of your hand. The point is just below your thumb, one thumb width under the crease of your wrist.
5–7 a.m.	LARGE INTESTINE 1	Look at the top of your hand; extend your index finger. The point is at the edge of your index finger's nailbed, on the side of the finger that rests alongside your thumb.
7–9 a.m.	STOMACH 36	Sit with your feet on the floor. Cup your palm just under your knee cap. The point is just below where your hand is resting, in a soft spot on the outer front of your shin.

JET LAG ACUPRESSURE CHART

Time at Destination	Name and Location of Point	How to Find the Point
9–11 a.m.	SPLEEN 3	From the arch side of your foot, locate the base of your big toe. The point rests on a soft hollow on the inside of the base of your big toe.
11 a.m.–1 p.m.	HEART 8	Look at the palm of your hand and make a fist. The point is where your little finger meets your palm.
1–3 p.m.	SMALL INTESTINE 5	Look at the palm of your hand; turn your hand slightly to focus on the side of your hand where your pinky finger rests. The point is on the edge of your wrist, in the depression where your hand and wrist meet, very close to the wrist crease.

JET LAG ACUPRESSURE CHART

Time at Destination	Name and Location of Point	How to Find the Point
3–5 p.m.	BLADDER 66	The point is on the outer side of the foot, where your little toe meets the rest of the foot
5–7 p.m.	KIDNEY 10	Sit with your feet flat on the floor. The point is near the bend of the knee between two tendons where the side and back of your leg meet.
7–9 p.m.	PERICARDIUM 8	Look at the palm of your hand and make a fist. The point is where your middle finger touches your palm.

JET LAG ACUPRESSURE CHART

Time at Destination	Name and Location of Point	How to Find the Point
9–11 p.m.	**TRIPLE WARMER 6**	Look at the top of your hand. The point is four fingers of width down from your wrist crease, in the middle of your forearm.
11 p.m.– 1 a.m.	**GALLBLADDER 41**	The point is on the top of your foot, midway between your ankle and the web of your little toe.
1–3 a.m.	**LIVER 1**	The point is on the top of your foot, at the base of the nail on your big toe that is closest to your second toe.

TECHNIQUE 23

Acupressure for Jet Lag

It would be so helpful if we could adjust instantaneously to the time change brought on by traveling across time zones. If only we could push a reset button, making our nervous system understand that we are suddenly shifting our daily routine to a different schedule. Then our jet-lag adjustment would be very smooth, or there would be no jet lag at all!

Resetting our internal clock is not as easy as we would like it to be; however, this technique will enable your body to speed up the process. By activating acupressure points on your head, you provide feedback to your brain and your pineal gland, the daily timekeepers of your central nervous system. This technique can help to "wake up" the circadian control centers to make faster accommodations.

For this jet-lag balancing technique, we make use of some of the points located on what's known as the "governing vessel meridian," one of two meridians that run along the center line of our bodies. Studies of anatomy have revealed the connection between this acupressure meridian and our central nervous system. Some of the acupressure points on this meridian are used to uplift our energy and our mood; they can make us more alert while calming us down at the same time.

HOW TO DO IT

1. Imagine a line drawn across the center of your head, starting in the middle of your front hairline, and then reaching over the top of your head toward the back of your hairline. The line should fall exactly down the middle of your head, as if you were parting your hair in the middle.

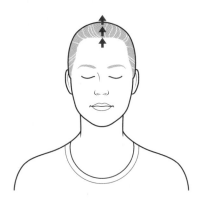

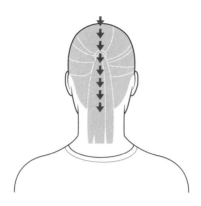

2. Put your fingertips (using everything except your thumb) on the beginning of this line, starting at the front of your hairline. Gently apply pressure with your fingertips, stimulating the acupressure points that are located along this center channel.

3. Move your fingertips back half an inch at a time and continue to press and stimulate the center meridian of your body. Work from the front of your head all the way to the back hairline by applying ample pressure for approximately ten to thirty seconds at each spot.

4. As always, listen to your body's needs as you gauge the appropriate amount of pressure to apply. You may feel some tenderness in certain areas, which is only an indication that your body is welcoming the balance you are creating through acupressure.

• • •

Part IV:

Theory and Background on the Techniques

The Art of Napping

"No day is so bad it can't be fixed with a nap."
—CARRIE SNOW

Cats know a thing or two about life. Not only have they been touted as Zen masters, knowing how to live in the moment, but they are also great nappers. We can learn a whole lot from them! Research has revealed some startling benefits to the midday snooze. While modern businesses are always looking for cutting-edge and high-tech solutions for the workplace that will help us do more with less, they might want to consider a different approach. Taking a nap at work might seem counterproductive, but what if it could actually *increase* productivity at the office?

Our bodies like getting an added twenty minutes of sleep during the day—much more so than adding twenty minutes to our total sleep time at night. A short twenty-minute nap has been proven to make us more alert, improve our mood, replenish our relaxation hormones, and pull us out of that all-dangerous "overdrive" mode. The stress hormone cortisol—

important when running away from a perceived danger like a saber-toothed tiger, but detrimental to our health in our modern-day life—is reduced or reined in, so to speak, during and as a result of a nap. That's why you may have noticed feeling much calmer after a few minutes of daytime z's.

Whether you had a good night's sleep or not, a nap can improve health, memory function, and mental performance. A 1995 NASA research study found that allowing pilots to take short naps during flights significantly increased alertness and reduced fatigue. The pilots who were not allowed to take naps had significantly more performance issues. If this is not convincing enough, know that napping also reduces mental overload and firms up your memory bank. You are more likely to remember learned material after a snooze. Last but not least, a nap improves your mood, which makes the latter part of your day more enjoyable.

As mentioned earlier in this book, some companies have introduced nap pods to some of their offices, allowing their employees to sneak in a little rest time during the day. Not only does it help their employees' stamina and mental performance, but it is reflected in their improved work performance.

The secret to a successful nap lies in its duration. While a long nap of an hour or two can cause grogginess, also called "sleep inertia," a twenty-minute nap will make you more alert, according to nap researchers. Considering that a nap can improve your health, relationship dynamics, mental alertness, work performance, and decision making, it seems like a winning proposition.

• • •

Reacquainting Yourself with Rest

There is nothing like sleep! Sleep rewires the nervous system, increases the function of the immune system, releases beneficial growth hormone, firms up our memory banks, and improves our mood, coping mechanisms, and productivity. During sleep, our brainwaves follow a specific pattern that is unmatched in any other physical state we're known to be in during the day or night. For example, the stages of deep sleep known as "REM-based dream sleep," which research shows we need to function at our best, cannot be accomplished in any other state—not even deeply restful states of meditation. However, that does not mean there are not benefits to rest. The body-mind needs both. It is important to distinguish between *sleep* and *rest,* and realize the benefits of what might be defined as a restful, quiet, and relaxed state of wakefulness.

A period of rest during the day is different than, let's say, a short nap at some point during your waking hours. According to sleep researcher and author Matthew Edlund, MD, sleep is not the only cure-all for the needs of our minds and bodies. Aside from the benefits that a sound sleep provides, a rest can have profound effects on our well-being, making us feel more connected to ourselves and the people around us. It is vital in enhancing our lives, life quality, and energy levels with measurable effects.

We have lost touch not only with healthy sleep patterns, but also with vital aspects of rest. We struggle to incorporate rest into our lives. Reviving the art of rest is beneficial to our overall sense of quality of life as well as our energy levels.

There are many ways to rest—it is more than just the state of "not doing." The list below will give you some insight into the different forms of rest and why they can be rejuvenating.

Passive Rest

When we think of resting, many things come to mind. There's the common notion of putting up our feet and relaxing on a couch, or shutting our eyes without actually falling asleep. Watching a movie, reading a book, or indulging in favorite snacks while lounging in a comfortable chair are all popular ways of resting. There is certainly a lot of value in this kind of physical relaxation, which is called a passive rest.

Social Rest

As humans, we have the need to feel socially connected. Socializing with friends, family members, and colleagues reduces depression and minimizes levels of the stress hormone cortisol. It has been shown to improve our heart health and recovery from illnesses. Chatting and connecting with fellow human beings is vital to a healthy lifestyle. Communicating with others balances hormones and neurotransmitters, and we can feel uplifted after just the right amount of social interaction that allows us to regroup and reconnect without feeling drained.

Mental Rest

We have become so accustomed to multitasking that many of us do not take the time to focus on just one activity wholeheartedly. We text while eating, talk on the phone while driving, and keep various trains of thought recirculating in our minds simultaneously. Getting a break from having too many mental irons in the fire and only concentrating on one thing at a time gives our nervous system a well-deserved holiday. Many of the techniques in this book help us focus on one thing at a time—a mindfulness approach that creates rest and relaxation. By resting your mind and only focusing on one thing, you feel more energetic and you can reconnect to your being. This also comes with the noted health benefits of a reduced heart rate and normalized blood pressure.

Creative Rest

As a child, you may have played in ways that allowed you to forget time and space around you. Do you manage to do the same as an adult? A creative rest allows you to tap into your creative potential—whatever form it takes—while forgetting your surroundings. It is deeply rejuvenating to your body, mind, and spirit. Whether knitting, drawing, painting fun designs on your fingernails, playing music, building sand castles, or making a new end table in your workshop, creative outlets are a holiday from our daily routine, chores, and busy minds. Such activities can de-stress and energize us.

Physical Rest

The art of physical rest may evoke various activities, depending on your preferences and resources. It may involve walking in nature, yoga and tai chi, or playing a few holes of golf. Any short-term physical activity that does not tire you can energize your body and mind, as well as make you feel more vibrant and alive.

The other day, my twenty-year-old daughter invited me to go rock climbing in the pristine nature of the Canadian Shield. As an upper-middle-aged woman, this was not a routine physical activity for me. With the able help of seasoned rock climbers, I climbed up a smooth rock cliff and had no choice but to focus on the task in front of me. Having to focus so completely, I realized I was getting a physical and mental rest. There was no option other than to pull my thoughts back from focusing on my fear of heights or worry about succeeding at an activity I'm not familiar with. The climbing was not a prolonged physical activity; rather, it was a twenty-minute adventure. The effect was a sense of rejuvenation. This kind of physical rest can contribute to better health and a stronger mind-body connection, and can provide all the benefits of deep, passive relaxation.

Spiritual Rest

A spiritual rest is the rejuvenating effect of spending some time in contemplation, meditation, or prayer.

Engaging in breathing exercises, reading spiritual scripts, pondering inspirational quotes, attending religious or spiritual services, and meditating all fall into this category of restful being and practice. Spiritual reconnection transforms our *doing* into a sense of deeper existence. Feeling connected with the deeper aspects of our being refocuses our priorities and helps us flow with *what is.* A spiritual practice helps us arrive at decisions in a more organic manner, rather than zapping our energy by rethinking the same thoughts over and over again. Zen and ancient Chinese masters would call this the "art of doing without doing," and research shows it aids in enhancing our mental, physical, and emotional health.

•

Deep, restful sleep is still the balm we need for our bodies, minds, and spirits. Sleep's health-promoting effects will not be accomplished merely by resting. However, combining a good night's sleep with a refreshing rest is undeniably helpful to our overall well-being.

• • •

The Organ Clock

We are very familiar with the internal rhythm of our bodies. Our "body clock" tells us when to eat, makes us tired at bedtime, and governs many important body functions—like digestion and the release of hormones. Our internal body clock rules over our body and organs, which is why our body-mind feels disoriented and confused when we travel and traverse time zones.

Traditional Chinese medicine explains that each energy meridian, and each organ in the body, has a specific two-hour interval of maximum activity each day. In other words, part of our circadian rhythm consists of energy flowing from one organ (or energy meridian) to another in two-hour intervals. The "organ clock" on the next page captures the meridian and organ activity across different times of the day.

While the paradigms of Eastern and Western medicine differ, there are many commonalities between the systems that enhance our understanding of the body. As an example, Western-trained physicians often find a correlation between the traditional

CHINESE ORGAN CLOCK

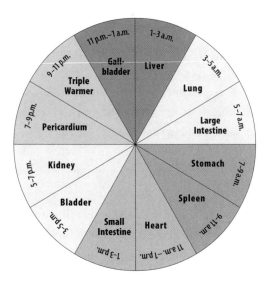

Chinese medicine organ clock and the physiology of our bodies. It is well known to on-call physicians in emergency rooms that, especially during certain types of weather conditions, incidents of severe asthma are more common between 3 and 5 a.m. According to the Chinese organ clock, that's the time of day in which lung energy is increased. As a matter of fact, on days when there are smog warnings, I have heard on-call physicians complain ahead of their night shifts that they would be unable to get a full night of sleep, as they knew that their asthma patients would require medical attention in the early morning hours during "lung time."

Another correlation is the late-afternoon slump, when we are overtaxed or have worked a full day. The 5 p.m. low we feel indicates that our adrenal/kidney energy needs a boost, as kidney time on the organ clock falls between 5 p.m. and 7 p.m.

Understanding the times of increased activity in specific meridians and organs can give us insight into helping ourselves. If you are prone to a 5 p.m. slump, you may want to consider a power nap after lunch. It most likely will help replenish some of your spent energy. Waking up in the middle of the night, at liver time, may mean that you need to be looking after your health and reducing your intake of substances that put stress on your liver. Water with a squeeze of lemon can be helpful in giving your liver some metabolic support. Planning and organizing in excess can also interfere with the optimum function of the liver, and you may want to adjust by exercising more and finding some relaxing leisure activities.

• • •

The Mechanics of Acupressure and the Meridian System

Acupressure and acupuncture make use of the body's meridian system, which was discovered a few thousand years ago by Chinese physicians. The meridian system is akin to the nervous system, but it is separate from the anatomical structures that we know in Western medicine.

Imagine twelve long, narrow "rivers" of energy flowing through either side of your body along prescribed paths. They are symmetrical, meaning they flow on each side of your body from head to toes and fingers, and vice versa. These rivers, or channels, of energy are important to our health in how they relate to our organs, other body parts, moods, and emotions.

We know that these channels, with about as many acupuncture points sprinkled on them as there are days in the year, carry an electrical charge that we can measure with an "ohmmeter," a device electricians use to measure electrical resistance. An acupuncture point conducts more electricity than its surrounding skin, and applying pressure to the point will help to balance this flow of electrical energy and create a self-healing response in your body.

Diagnosis in Chinese Medicine

In ancient China, autopsies were forbidden and medicine became the subtle art of "listening" to the body. Chinese doctors were trained to be very observant and fine-tuned in the art of assessing their patients. There are three major ways that specialists of Chinese medicine find out what is going on in the body: namely, taking a careful history, taking the pulse in a way unique to this discipline, and looking at the tongue.

The first method is obvious and is used in any type of medicine. The patient reports as exactly as possible what he or she experiences in the body and mind; the aches and pains; and particular circumstances, patterns, and time frames of the complaints. The second method, taking the pulse, is a way of discovering what is going on inside the body by taking several pulses on both wrists. Chinese pulse diagnosis offers a window into the function of organ systems without blood work, lab tests, and imaging. It takes many years of practice and learning to perfect the art and interpretation of "pulse diagnosis."

A number of years ago, I traveled to China to study medical Qigong, an ancient system of postures, movements, and meditation techniques to create mind-body harmony. We visited a traditional Chinese medicine hospital and underwent Chinese pulse diagnosis performed by doctors on staff. The diagnosis established by these doctors, who knew nothing about our medical history, was astounding. They accurately described symptoms, imbalances, and illnesses in many of us.

When I learned the art of Chinese medicine at a course in Toronto, our teacher had us practice pulse diagnosis on other students. As I was feeling the pulse position relating to the heart, I noticed a "weak" pulse wave under the tip of my finger. The student, an upper-middle-aged man, confirmed that he had had a heart attack a couple of years previously. It seemed almost eerie to me then, but this kind of experience has become commonplace to me now after practicing Chinese medicine for more than two decades.

In addition to history taking and pulse diagnosis, Chinese medicine specialists practice the art of tongue diagnosis. The color, shape, and size of the tongue reveal much about a person's state of health and the condition of his or her specific meridians.

These three diagnostic tools give the doctors the information required to assess the meridian system and treat their patients. It is an eye-opening experience to have a doctor who is well trained in Chinese medicine and pulse diagnosis tell you about your state of health on a mental, emotional, and physical level without even knowing your name or your health history.

•

Famous Canadian neurophysiologist Dr. Bruce Pomeranz has conducted extensive research on how acupuncture affects the meridian system and found that potent neurotransmitters are released that benefit the body's healing system. This research is very important and meaningful; it does not, however, explain exactly why stimulating very specific acupressure points can help to treat certain illnesses and support the health of an individual. Therefore, if you decide that you would like to explore using acupuncture or acupressure to treat a specific condition beyond the techniques in this book, finding a well-trained practitioner will make all the difference.

• • •

Resources

Websites

Centers for Disease Control and Prevention. "Behavioral Risk Factor Surveillance System: 2015 BRFSS Survey Data and Documentation." Last modified September 15, 2016. www.cdc.gov/brfss /annual_data/annual_2015.html.

CNBC. "Why Aetna's CEO pays workers up to $500 to sleep." CNBC. April 5, 2016. www.cnbc.com /2016/04/05/why-aetnas-ceo-pays-workers-up-to -500-to-sleep.html.

Rosekind, Mark R., David F. Dinges, Linda J. Connell, Michael S. Rountree, Cheryl L. Spinweber, and Kelly A. Gillen. "Crew Factors in Flight Operations IX: Effects of Planned Cockpit Rest on Crew Performance and Alertness in Long-Haul Operations." NASA *Technical Memorandum* 108839 (Sept. 1994): 51–4. https://ntrs.nasa.gov /archive/nasa/casi.ntrs.nasa.gov/19950006379.pdf.

Rosekind, Mark. "The Science of Sleep." Common Ground Speaker Series, January 30, 2014. www .commongroundspeakerseries.org/wp-content/ uploads/2014/07/RosekindSummary.pdf.

Books

Edlund, Matthew. *The Power of Rest: Why Sleep Alone Is Not Enough.* San Francisco: HarperOne, 2010.

Gach, Michael Reed. *Acupressure's Potent Points.* New York: Bantam, 1990.

Gerber, Richard. *Vibrational Medicine: The #1 Handbook of Subtle-Energy Therapies.* 3rd edition. Rochester, VT: Bear and Company, 2001.

Tolle, Eckhart. *The Power of Now: A Guide to Spiritual Enlightenment.* Vancouver, BC: Namaste Publishing, 2004.

• • •

Acknowledgments

My deep gratitude to the amazing publishing team at Hazelden Publishing. Working with my editor Vanessa Torrado and production manager Heather Silsbee, as well as the many skilled and able professionals at Hazelden Publishing, was a delight. I am grateful for the opportunity to publish more self-help techniques for the benefit of the readers. A special thank you to my clients and friends who willingly contributed to this book in countless ways.

• • •

About the Author

Katrin Schubert has dedicated her career to helping her fellow human beings heal their bodies, minds, and spirits with natural medicine. After completing her medical degree and a PhD in 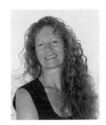 human genetics at the University of Hamburg, and receiving international training in England, the Czech Republic, India, China, Canada, and the United States, she opened her holistic health clinics in Kingston and Gananoque, Ontario, Canada. Katrin also has a science degree from Queen's University in Kingston. She is the author of the first two books in the 5-Minute First Aid for the Mind series, *Relieve Stress* and *Reduce Craving*. You can contact Katrin through her website: www.drkatrin.com.

About Hazelden Publishing

As part of the Hazelden Betty Ford Foundation, Hazelden Publishing offers both cutting-edge educational resources and inspirational books. Our print and digital works help guide individuals in treatment and recovery, and their loved ones. Professionals who work to prevent and treat addiction also turn to Hazelden Publishing for evidence-based curricula, digital content solutions, and videos for use in schools, treatment programs, correctional programs, and electronic health records systems. We also offer training for implementation of our curricula.

Through published and digital works, Hazelden Publishing extends the reach of healing and hope to individuals, families, and communities affected by addiction and related issues.

For more information about Hazelden publications,
please call **800-328-9000**
or visit us online at **hazelden.org/bookstore**.